CNA Study Guide

Julie Johnson RN, MSN

ISBN-13: 978-1500678487

ISBN-10: 1500678481

ISBN-13: 978-1497343122

ISBN-10: 1497343127

Printed in the United States of America.

Dedication

To all Nurse Assistant Students

In this book, you will review:

The Medical History

Vital Signs

Patient Care Positions

Safety in the Healthcare Environment

Infection Control

Section One

General Information For The Nurse Assistants

Nurse Assistants, also known as nursing aides, geriatric aides, unlicensed assistive personnel, or hospital attendants, perform routine tasks under the supervision of nursing and medical staff. They answer patients' call lights, deliver messages, serve meals, make beds, and help patients eat, dress, and bathe. CNAs also may provide skin care to patients; take their temperatures, pulse rate, respiration rate, and blood pressure; and help patients get in and out of bed and walk. They also may escort patients to operating and examining rooms, keep patients' rooms neat, set up equipment, store and move supplies, or assist with some procedures. They observe patients' physical, mental, and emotional conditions and report any change to the nursing or medical staff.

CNAs help care for physically or mentally ill, injured, disabled, or infirm individuals confined to hospitals, nursing care facilities, and mental health settings. Home health aides' duties are similar, but they work in patients' homes or residential care facilities.

This is usually an entry level for individuals who wish to become nurses in the future. Students are taught principles of infection control, communication techniques, and the skills to safely care for people. These skills include bathing, dressing, assisting to eat, grooming, toileting, lifting and moving while using proper body mechanics.

Upon completion of the nurse assistant training course, students will be able to:

Technical Skills

- Demonstrate awareness of industry standards.
- Define Title 22 regulations regarding the rights of patients.
- Follow hospital safety rules; discuss the role of a nurse assistant in an emergency.

- Practice proper use of body mechanics and positioning techniques using devises for patient comfort and safety.

- Practice centigrade and Fahrenheit conversions for weight, length and liquid volume.

- Demonstrate ability to bathe, dress, and perform personal hygiene tasks for patients.

- Demonstrate ability to collect specimens, remove urinary catheters, apply dressings and make beds.

- Take temperature, pulse and respiration; take accurate blood pressure; document findings.

- Distinguish between types of diet therapies; serve and feed patients.

- Recognize signs and symptoms of distress; react and intervene appropriately.

- Demonstrate ability to care for patients with neurological disorders and aged residents.

- Assist patient with rehabilitative processes and with activities of daily living.

Personal and Professional Skills

- Discuss disinfection and sterilization, hazardous waste disposal, and standard precautions.

- Demonstrate effective patient care documentation.

- Discuss stages of dying and related care; interaction with families; and post-mortem care.

- Demonstrate appropriate work ethics and professional demeanor as demanded by the industry.

- Demonstrate the ability to work independently or as a member of a team.

- Listen attentively, follow directions and effectively relay directions to others.

Career Planning Skills

- Research career opportunities; establish educational and career goals related to the health care industry.

- Research employment opportunities; prepare a resume; prepare for an interview.

WORKING CONDITIONS

Most full-time patient care technicians work about 40 hours a week. However, since some patients need care 24 hours a day, some CNAs work evenings, nights, weekends, and holidays. Many work part time. Nurse Assistants spend many hours standing and walking, and they often face heavy workloads. Because they may have to move patients in and out of bed or help them stand or walk, aides must guard against back injury. CNAs also may face hazards from minor infections and major diseases, such as hepatitis, but can avoid infections by following proper procedures.

CNAs often have unpleasant duties, such as emptying bedpans and changing soiled bed linens. The patients they care for may be disoriented, irritable, or uncooperative. While their work can be emotionally demanding, many CNAs gain satisfaction from assisting those in need.

JOB OUTLOOK

Numerous job openings for patient care technicians will arise from a combination of fast employment growth and high replacement needs. High replacement needs in this large occupation reflect modest entry requirements, low pay, high physical and emotional demands, and lack of opportunities for advancement. For these same reasons, many people are unwilling to perform the kind of work required by the occupation. Therefore, persons who are interested in, and suited for, this work should have excellent job opportunities.

Overall employment of patient care technicians is projected to grow for all occupations through the year 2020, although individual occupational growth rates will vary. Employment of CNAs is expected to grow the fastest, as a result of both growing demand for home healthcare services from an aging population and efforts to contain healthcare costs by moving patients out of hospitals and nursing care facilities as quickly as possible. Consumer preference for care in the home and improvements in medical technologies for in-home treatment also will contribute to faster-than-average employment growth for CNAs and HHAs.

The Medical History

Parts of the patient's medical history are:

-Chief complaint (CC): the reason why the patient came to see the physician.

- History of present illness (HPI): this is an explanation of the chief complaint

to determine the onset of the illness; associated symptoms; what the patient

has done to treat the condition, etc.

-Past, Family and Social History (PFSH):

- Past medical history: includes all health problems, major illnesses,

surgeries the patient has had, current medications complete with reasons

for taking them, and allergies.

- Family history: summary of health problems of siblings, parents, and other

blood relatives that could alert the physician to hereditary and/or familial

diseases.

-Social history: includes marital status, occupation, educational attainment,

hobbies, use of alcohol, tobacco, drugs, and lifestyles.

-Review of Systems - this is an orderly and systematic check of each organ and

system of the body by questions. Both positive and pertinent negative

findings are documented. The ROS, in conjunction with the physical examination, helps elicit

information that is essential to the diagnosis of patient's condition.

Vital Signs

Reflect the functions of three body processes necessary for life:

Body temperature

Respiration

Heart function

The four vital signs of body function are:

Temperature

Pulse

Respiration

Blood pressure

Temperature

Body temperature is a balance between heat production and heat loss in conjunction with each other, maintained and regulated by the hypothalamus.

Thermometers are used to measure temperature using the Fahrenheit and Centigrade or Celsius scale. Temperature sites are the following: mouth, rectum, ear (tympanic membrane), and the axilla (underarm). The normal ranges for each site are:

Site	Normal Range
Rectal	98.6Fto 100.6F (37.0C to 38.1C)
Oral	97.6F to 99.6F (36.5C to 37.5C)
Axillary	96.6F to 98.6F (35.9C to 37.0C)
Tympanic Membrane	98.6F (37C)

Some terms used to describe body temperature are:

Febrile – presence of fever

Afebrile – absence of fever

Fever – elevated body temperature beyond normal range. Types of fever are:

Intermittent: fluctuating fever that returns to or below baseline then rises again.

Remittent: fluctuating fever that remains elevated; it does not return to baseline temperature.

Continuous: a fever that remains constant above the baseline; it does not fluctuate.

Oral temperature is the most common method of measurement; however, it is not taken from the following patients:

- infants and children less than six years old

- patients who has had surgery or facial, neck, nose, or mouth injury

- those receiving oxygen

- those with nasogastric tubes

- patients with convulsive seizure

- hemiplegic patients

- patients with altered mental status

Wait for 30 minutes to take the oral temperature in patients who have just finished eating, drinking, or smoking. When taking the temperature, leave the thermometer in the patient's mouth for 3-5 minutes or as required by agency policy.

Rectal temperature is taken when oral temperature is not feasible. However, it is not taken from the following patients:

- patients with heart disease

- patients with rectal disease or disorder or has had rectal surgery

- patients with diarrhea

It is taken with the patient in a side-lying position and the thermometer and the patient's hip is held throughout the procedure so the thermometer is not lost in the rectum or broken.

Axillary temperature is the least accurate and is taken only when no other temperature site can be used. The axilla, (the underarm) should be clean and dry and the thermometer should be held in place for 5-10 minutes or as required by the facility policy.

Tympanic temperature is useful for children and confused patients because of the speed of operation of the tympanic thermometer. A covered probe is gently inserted into the ear canal and temperature is measured within seconds (1–3 seconds). It is not used if the patient has an ear disorder or ear drainage.

Pulse

The normal adult pulse rate ranges between 60 and 100 beats per minute. The site most commonly used for taking pulse is the radial artery found in the wrist on the same side as the thumb. It is felt with the first two or three fingers (never with the thumb) and usually taken for 30 seconds multiplied by two to get the rate per minute. If the rate is unusually fast or slow, however, count it for 60 seconds.

The apical pulse is a more accurate measurement of the heart rate and it is taken over the apex of the heart by auscultation using the stethoscope. It is used for patients with irregular heart rate and for infants and small children.

Respiration

When measuring respiration, respiratory characteristics such as rate, rhythm, and depth are taken into account. Rate is the number of respirations per minute. The normal range for adults is 12 to 20 per minute. One inspiration (inhale) and one expiration (exhale) counts as one respiration. It is counted for 30 seconds multiplied by two or for a full minute.

Some rate abnormalities are the following:

Apnea – this is a temporary complete absence of breathing which may be a result of a reduction in the stimuli to the respiratory centers of the brain.

Tachypnea – this is a respiration rate of greater than 40/min. It is transient in the newborn and maybe caused by the hysteria in the adult.

Bradypnea – decrease in numbers of respirations. This occurs during sleep. It may also be due to certain diseases. Respiratory rhythm refers to the pattern of breathing. It can vary with age: infants have an irregular rhythm while adults have regular.

Some abnormalities in the rhythm are the following:

Cheyne-Stokes – this is a regular pattern of irregular breathing rate.

Orthopnea – this is difficulty or inability to breath unless in an upright position.

Depth of respiration refers to the amount of air that is inspired and expired during each respiration. Some abnormalities in the depth of respirations are the following:

Hypoventilation: state in which reduced amount of air enters the lungs resulting in decreased oxygen level and increased carbon dioxide level in blood. It can be due to breathing that is too shallow, or too slow, or to diminished lung function.

Hyperpnea: abnormal increase in the depth and rate of breathing.

Hyperventilation: state in which there is an increased amount of air entering the lungs.

Blood Pressure

This is the measurement of the amount of force exerted by the blood on the peripheral arterial walls and is expressed in millimeters (mm) of mercury (Hg).The measurement consist of two components: the highest (systole) and lowest (diastole) amount of pressure exerted during the cardiac cycle.

A stethoscope and sphygmomanometer of either aneroid or mercury type are used. The size of the cuff of the sphygmomanometer will depend on the circumference of the limb and not the age of the patient. The width of the inflatable bag within the cuff should be about 40% of this circumference – 12 cm to 14 cm in an average adult. The length of the bag should be about 80% of this circumference – almost long enough to encircle the arm. Cuffs that are too short or narrow may give falsely high readings, e.g. a regular cuff on an obese arm may lead to a false diagnosis of hypertension.

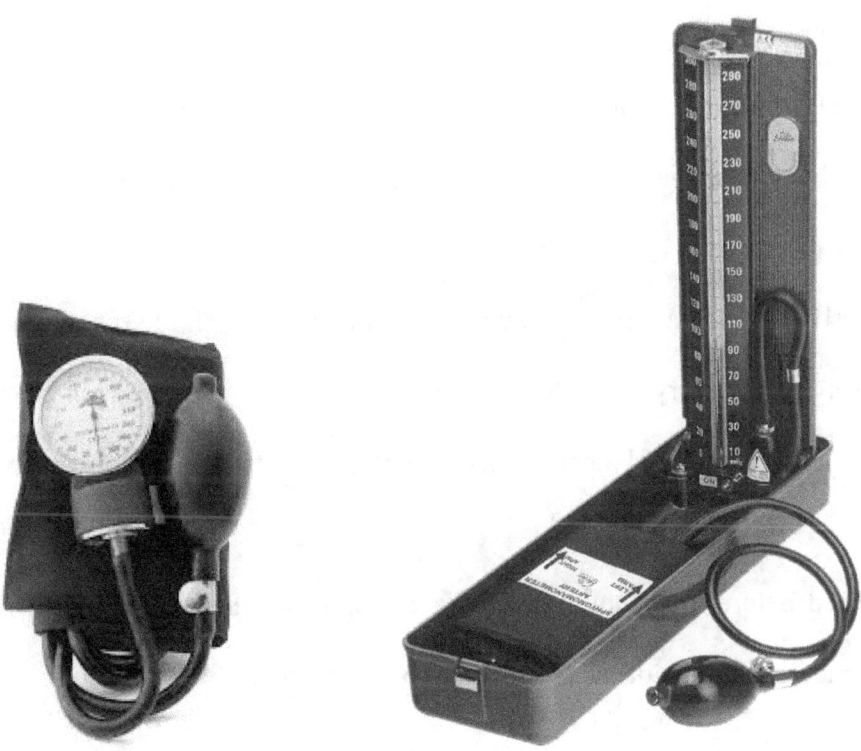

The inflatable bag is centered over the brachial artery with the lower border about 2.5cm above the antecubital crease. The cuff is positioned at heart level. If the brachial artery is far below the heart level the blood pressure will appear falsely high. If the brachial artery is far above heart level, blood pressure will appear falsely low.

Blood pressure is taken by determining first the palpatory systolic pressure over the brachial artery. Then with the bell of the stethoscope over the brachial artery, the cuff is inflated again to about 30 mm Hg above the palpatory systolic pressure and deflated slowly, allowing the pressure to drop at a rate of about 2 to 3 mmHg per second. Note the level at which you hear the sounds of at least two consecutive beats. This is the systolic pressure. Continue to lower the pressure slowly until the sounds become muffled and then disappear. Then deflate the cuff rapidly to zero. The disappearance point, which is usually only a few mmHg below the muffling point, marks the generally accepted diastolic pressure. Both the systolic and diastolic pressure levels are read the nearest 2 mmHg.

Common errors in blood pressure measurements:

Improper cuff size. Cuffs that are too short or narrow may give falsely high readings. Using a regular cuff on an obese arm may lead to a false diagnosis of hypertension. For an obese arm, select a cuff with a larger than standard bag.

The arm is not at heart level. If the brachial artery is much below the heart level, the blood pressure will appear falsely high. Conversely, if the artery is much above heart level, blood pressure will appear falsely low. A 13.6 cm difference between arterial and cardiac levels produces a blood pressure error of 10mmHg.

Cuff is not completely deflated before use. Deflation of the cuff is faster than 2-3 mmHg per second. Rapid deflation will lead to underestimation of the systolic and overestimation of the diastolic

pressure.

The cuff is re-inflated during the procedure without allowing the arm to rest for 1-2 minute between readings. Repetitive inflation of the cuff can result in venous congestion, which could make the sound less audible producing artifactually low systolic and high diastolic pressure.

Improper cuff placement.

Defective equipment. A bag that balloons outside the cuff leads to falsely high readings.

Anthropometric Measurements

The term anthropometric refers to comparative measurements of the body. They are used as indicators of the state of health and well-being of the patient and are often included in the initial measurement of vital signs. Anthropometric measurements require precise measuring techniques to be valid.

Length, height, weight, weight-for-length, and head circumference (length is used in infants and toddlers, rather than height, because they are unable to stand) are used to assess growth and development in infants, children and adolescents. Individual measurements are usually compared to reference standards on a growth chart.

Height, weight, body mass index (BMI), waist-to-hip ratio, and percentage of body fat are the measurements used for adults. These measures are then compared to reference standards to assess weight status and the risk for various diseases.

Patient Care Positions

Positioning a Patient for Examination or Treatment

When performing an examination, treatment, tests or to obtain specimens, patients are put in special positions.

The Horizontal Recumbent Position is used for most physical examinations. The patient lies on his/her back with legs extended. Arms may be above the head, alongside the body or folded on the chest.

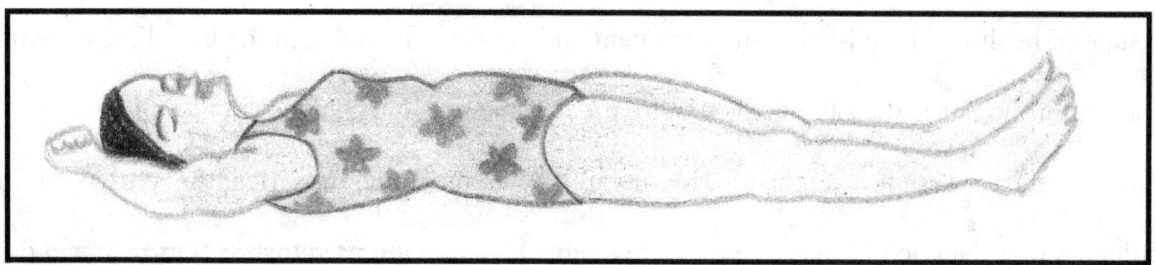

Figure 1-1. Horizontal recumbent position.

The Dorsal Recumbent Position is when the patient is on his/her back with knees flexed and soles of the feet flat on the bed. The PCT will need to fold a sheet once across the chest and fold a second sheet crosswise over the thighs and legs so that genital area is easily exposed.

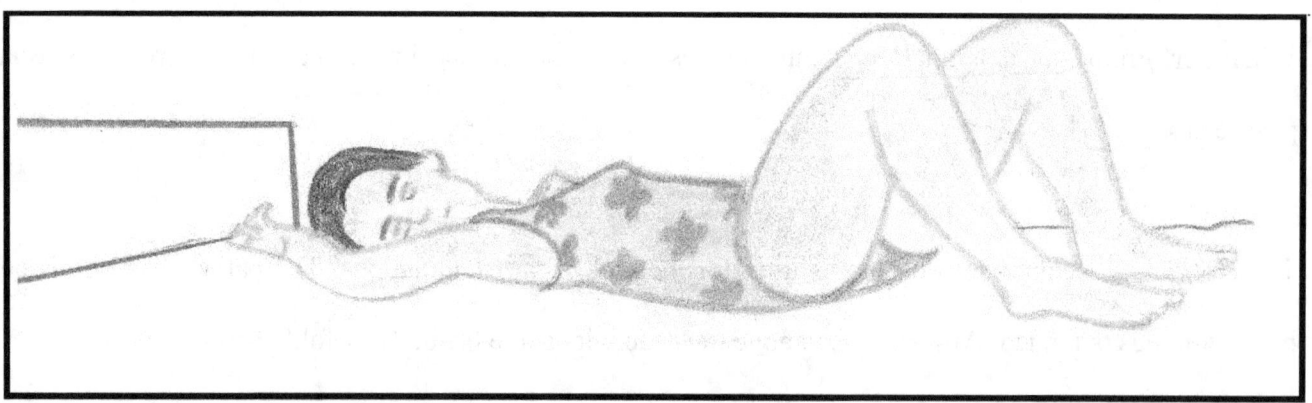

Figure 1-2. Dorsal recumbent position

The Fowler's Position is used to promote drainage or to ease breathing. A sitting or semi-sitting position where the back of the examination table is elevated to either 45 degrees (Semi-Fowler's) or 90 degrees (High- Fowler's). The knees maybe raised slightly by placing a pillow underneath, but usually the legs rest flat on the table. . The patient may need a foot support. This position is usually used for patients with cardiovascular or respiratory problems, and for the examination of the upper body and head.

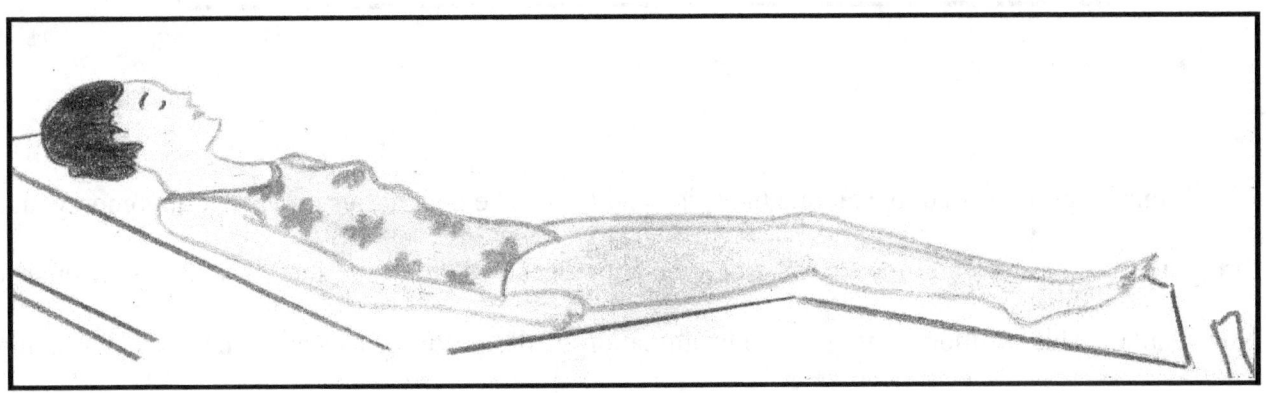

Figure 1-3. Fowler's position.

The Dorsal Lithotomy Position is used for examination of pelvic organs. This position is similar to the dorsal recumbent position, except that the patient's legs are well separated and thighs are acutely flexed. The feet are usually placed in stirrups and a folded sheet or bath blanket is placed crosswise over thighs and legs so that genital area is easily exposed. Keep the patient covered as much as possible.

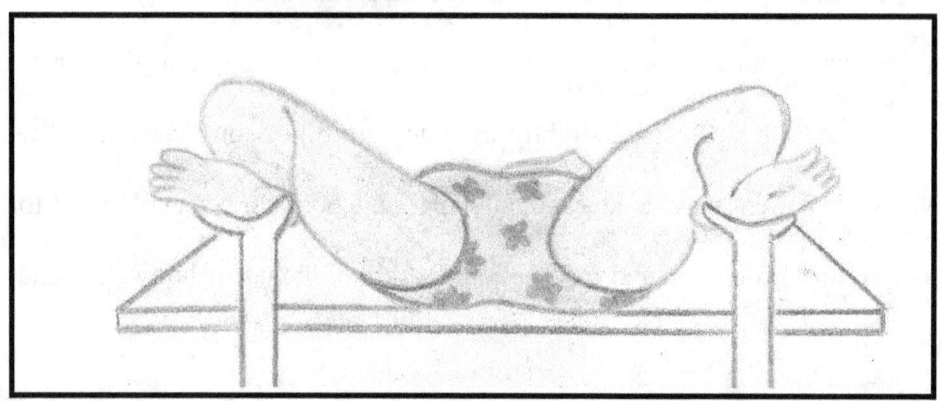

The Prone Position is used to examine the spine and back. The patient lies on his/her abdomen with head turned to one side for comfort, the arms may be above head or alongside the body. Cover with sheet or bath blanket. This position is used in the examination of the posterior aspect of the body, including the back or spine. NOTE: An unconscious patient or one with an abdominal incision or breathing difficulty usually cannot lie in this position.

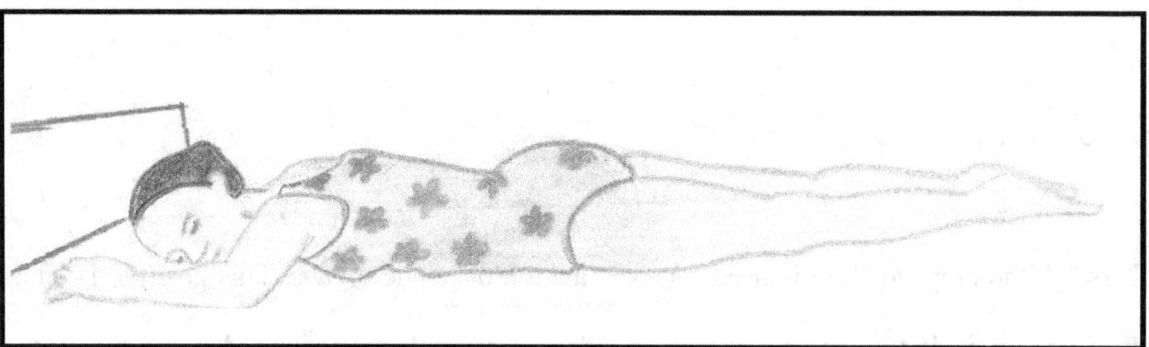

Figure 1-5. Prone position.

The Sim's Position is used for rectal examination. The patient is on his/her left side with the right knee flexed against the abdomen and the left knee slightly flexed. The left arm is behind the body; the right arm is placed comfortably. NOTE: Patient with leg injuries or arthritis usually cannot assume this position.

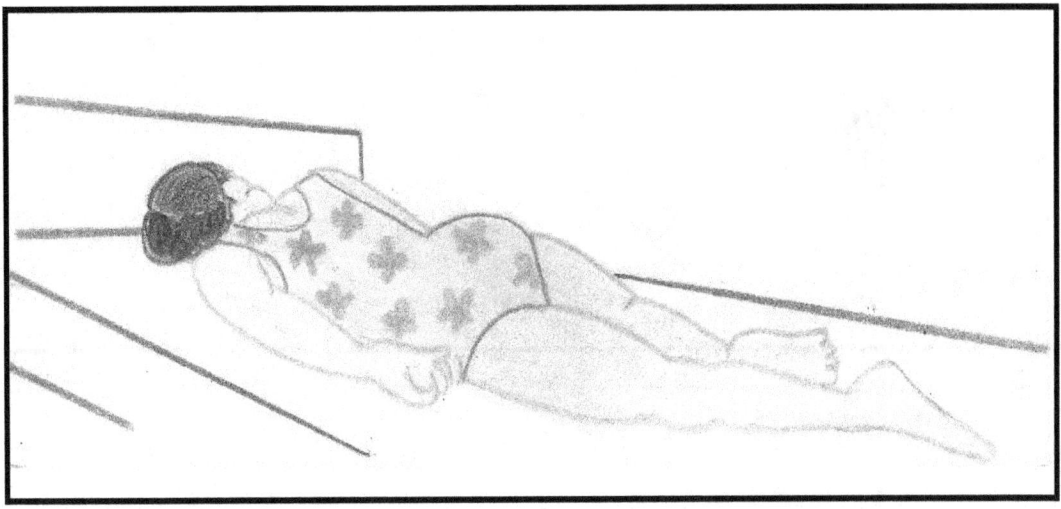

Figure 1-6. Sim's position.

The Knee-Chest Position is used for rectal and vaginal examinations and as treatment to bring the uterus into normal position. The patient is on his/her knees with his/her chest resting on the bed and elbows resting on the bed or arms above head. The head is turned to one side. The thighs are straight and lower legs are flat on the bed. NOTE: Do not leave patient alone; he/she may become dizzy, faint, and fall.

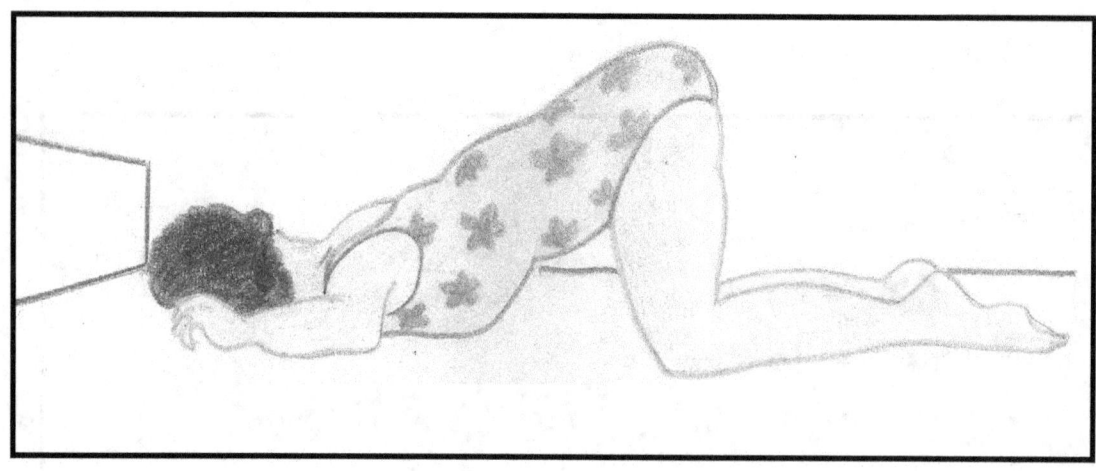

Figure 1-7. Knee-chest position.

Trendelenburg position – The patient is placed flat on the back, face up, the knees flexed and legs hanging off the end of the table, with the legs and feet supported by a footboard. The table is positioned with the head 45 degrees lower than the body. This position is used primarily for surgical procedures of pelvis and abdomen.

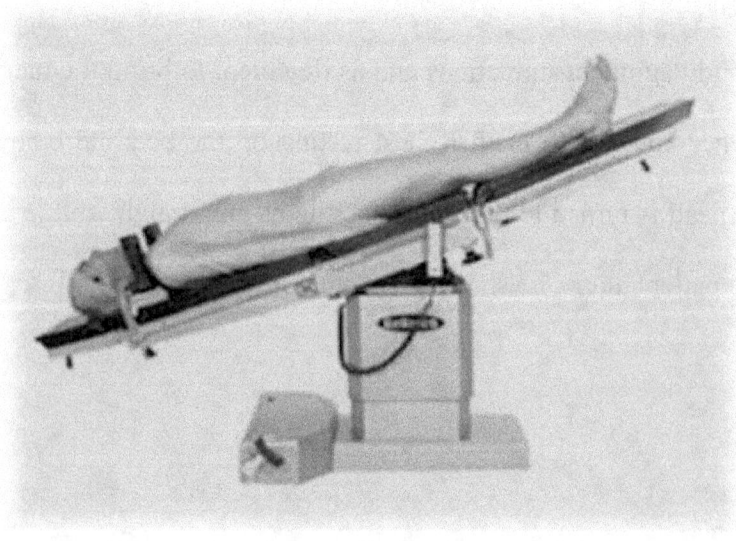

Safety

Safety hazards abound in the healthcare setting, many of which can cause serious injury or disease. The Occupational Safety and Health Administration (OSHA) is responsible for the identification of the various hazards present in the workplace and for the creation of rules and regulations to minimize exposure to such hazards. Employers are mandated to institute measures that will assure safe working conditions and health workers have the obligation to know and follow those measures.

Safety rules are usually based on common sense. Most accidents occur when these rules are neglected, overlooked or ignored. Accidents generally occur when safety is compromised because of haste and secondary shortcuts. These shortcuts can lead to personal injury and equipment damage. When an accident occurs, it must be reported to your supervisor immediately. Trying to cover up the incident can lead to serious, even disastrous results.

Hazards

A. Physical Hazards

Electrical Safety Regulations

Use only ground plugs that have been approved by Underwriters' Laboratory (UL).

Never use extension cords.

Avoid electrical circuit overloading.

Inspect all cords and plugs periodically for damage.

Use a surge protector on all sensitive electronic devices.

Before servicing, UNPLUG the device from the electrical outlet.

Use signs and/or labels to indicate high voltage or electrical hazards.

B. Chemical Hazards

Chemical Safety Regulations

If the skin or eyes come in contact with any chemicals, immediately wash the area with water for at least 5 minutes.

Store flammable or volatile chemicals in a well-ventilated area.

After use, immediately recap all bottles containing toxic substances.

Label all chemicals with the required Material Safety Data Sheet (MDSD) information.

C. Biological Hazards

Biological Safety Regulations

1. Disinfect the laboratory work area before and after each use when dealing with biologicals.

2. Never draw a specimen through a pipette by mouth. This technique is not permitted in the laboratory.

3. Always wear gloves.

4. Sterilize specimens and any other contaminated materials and/or dispose of them through incineration.

5. Wash hands thoroughly before and after every procedure.

Emergency First Aid

The ability to recognize and react quickly to an emergency may be the difference of life or death for the patient. As patients react differently to various situations, it is important for all healthcare professionals to be prepared in an emergency.

External Hemorrhage: controlling the bleeding is most effectively accomplished by elevating the affected part above heart level and applying direct pressure to the wound. Do not attempt to elevate a broken extremity   as   this   could   cause   further   damage.
Shock occurs when there is _insufficient return of blood flow to the heart, resulting in inadequate supply

of oxygen to all organs and tissues of the body.' Patients experiencing trauma may go into shock and for some patients, seeing their own blood may induce shock.

Common symptoms:

-Pale, cold, clammy skin

-Rapid, weak pulse

- Increased, shallow breathing rate

- Expressionless face/staring eyes.

First Aid for Shock:

-Maintain an open airway for the victim

-Call for assistance

-Keep the victim lying down with the head lower than the rest of the body

-Attempt to control bleeding or cause of shock (if known)

-Keep the victim warm until help arrives

Cardiopulmonary Resuscitation. Most healthcare institutions require their professionals to be certified in CPR. It is important for all professionals to maintain all certifications acquired.

Infection Control/Chain of Infection

This consists of links, each of which is necessary for the infectious disease to spread. Infection control is based on the fact that the transmission of infectious diseases will be prevented or stopped when any level in the chain is broken or interrupted.

Agent -------------- Mode of transmission ------------ Susceptible host

: :

: :

 portal of exit portal of entry

Agents– are infectious microorganisms that can be classified into groups namely: viruses, bacteria, fungi, and parasites. When infectious diseases are identified according to the specific disease-causing microorganism, the disease may be prevented with the use of anti-infective drugs or infection control practices.

Portal of exit –the method by which an infectious agent leaves its reservoir. Standard

Precautions and Transmission-Based Precautions are control measures aimed at

preventing the spread of the disease as infectious agents exit the reservoir.

Mode of transmission –specific ways in which microorganisms travel from the reservoir

to the susceptible host. There are five main types of mode of transmission:

- Contact : direct and indirect

- Droplet

- Airborne

- Common vehicle

- Vectorborne

Portal of entry – allows the infectious agent access to the susceptible host. Common

entry sites are broken skin, mucous membranes, and body systems exposed to the external environment such as the respiratory, gastrointestinal, and reproductive. Methods such as sterile wound care, transmission-based precautions, and aseptic technique limit the transmission of the infectious agents.

Susceptible host – The infectious agent enters a person who is not resistant or immune.

Control at this level is directed towards the identification of the patients at risk, treat their underlying condition for susceptibility, or isolate them from the reservoir.

Medical Asepsis

Best defined as —the destruction of pathogenic microorganisms after they leave the body.‖ It also involves environmental hygiene measures such as equipment cleaning and disinfection procedures. Methods of medical asepsis are Standard Precautions and

Transmission-Based Precautions

Disinfection. This procedure used in medical asepsis using various chemicals that can be used to destroy many pathogenic microorganisms. Since chemicals can irritate skin and mucous membranes, they are used only on inanimate objects.

The least expensive and most readily available disinfectant for surfaces such as

countertops is a 1:10 solution of household bleach. Boiling water (temperature of 212 F)

is considered a form of disinfection, but use of it in today‘s medical setting is limited to

items that:

1. will not be used in invasive procedures;

2. will not be inserted into body orifices nor be used in a sterile procedure

Surgical Asepsis

All microbial life, pathogens and nonpathogens, are destroyed before an invasive procedure is performed. Surgical asepsis and sterile technique are often used interchangeably.

Four methods of sterilization

1. Gas sterilization: often used for wheelchairs and hospital beds. Useful in hospitals, but costly for the office.

2. Dry heat sterilization: requires higher temperature that steam sterilization but longer exposure times. Used for instruments that easily corrodes.

3. Chemical sterilization - uses the same chemical used for chemical disinfection, but the exposure time is longer.

4. Steam sterilization (autoclave) - uses steam under pressure to obtain high temperature of 250-254F with exposure times of 20-40 minutes depending on the item being sterilized.

Handwashing

Hand washing is the most important means of preventing the spread of infection. A routine hand wash procedure uses plain soap to remove soil and transient bacteria. Hand antisepsis requires the use of antimicrobial soap to remove, kill or inhibit transient microorganisms. It is important that all healthcare personnel learn proper hand washing procedures.

Barrier Protection

Protective clothing provides a barrier against infection. Used properly, it will provide protection to the person wearing it; disposed of properly it will assist in the spread of infection. Learning how to put on and remove protective clothing is vital to insure the health and wellness of the person wearing the PPE. PPE's or personal protective equipment includes:

Masks

Goggles

Face Shields

Respirator

Isolation Precautions

For many years, the CDC recommended universal precautions, which is a method of infection control that assumed that all human blood and body fluids were potentially infectious. The CDC issued a revised guidelines consisting of two tiers or levels of precautions: Standard Precautions and Transmission-Based Precautions.

Standard Precautions

This is an infection control method designed to prevent direct contact with blood and other body fluids and tissues by using barrier protection and work control practices.

Under the standard precautions, all patients are presumed to be infective for blood-borne pathogens. Infection control practices to be used with all patients. These replace universal precautions and body substance isolation. They are used when there is a possibility of contact with any of the following:

- Blood

- All body fluids, secretions, and excretions (except sweat), regardless of whether or not they contain visible blood

- Nonintact skin

- Mucous membranes designed to reduce the risk of transmission of microorganisms from both

- Recognized and unrecognized sources of infections.

The standard precautions are:

Wear gloves when collecting and handling blood, body fluids, or tissue specimen.

Wear face shields when there is a danger for splashing on mucous membranes.
Dispose of all needles and sharp objects in puncture-proof containers without
recapping.

Transmission- Based Precautions the second tier of precautions and are to be used
when the patient is known or suspected of being infected with contagious disease. They
are to be used in addition to standard precautions. All types of isolation are condensed
into three categories:

Contact precautions: are designed to reduce the risk of transmission of microorganisms by direct or
indirect contact. Direct-contact transmission involves skin-to-skin contact and physical transfer of
microorganisms to a susceptible host from an infected or colonized person. Indirect-contact
transmission involves contact with a contaminated intermediate object in the
patient's environment.

Airborne precautions: are designed to reduce the risk of airborne transmission of infectious agents.
Microorganisms carried in this manner can be dispersed widely by air currents and may become inhaled
by or deposited on a susceptible host within the same room or over a longer distance from the source
patient. Special air handling and ventilation are required to prevent airborne transmission.
Contact precautions: are designed to reduce the risk of transmission of microorganisms by direct or
indirect contact. Direct-contact transmission involves skin-to-skin contact and physical transfer of
microorganisms to a susceptible host from an infected or colonized person. Indirect-contact
transmission involves contact with a contaminated intermediate object in the patient's environment.

Airborne precautions: are designed to reduce the risk of airborne transmission of infectious agents.
Microorganisms carried in this manner can be dispersed widely by air currents and may become inhaled
by or deposited on a susceptible host within the same room or over a longer distance from the source

patient. Special air handling and ventilation are required to prevent airborne transmission.

Section One Questions
1. Which of the following is an example of the duties of a nurse assistant?
   a. Handling basic paperwork
   b. Taking the vital signs of the patients
   c. Assisting in bed bath
   d. All of the above are functions of a CNA

2. What is a thermometer used for?
   a. Assessing the pulse of a patient
   b. Measuring blood pressure of a patient
   c. Measuring body temperature
   d. Assessing the responsiveness of a patient

3. An oral thermometer produces a reading of 101 degrees Fahrenheit. This patient is:
   a. Febrile
   b. Afebrile
   c. Normal
   d. None of the above

4. A fever that remains constant is:
   a. Remittent
   b. Afebrile
   c. Continuous
   d. Intermittent

5. Who should have their temperatures taken orally?
   a. Elderly patients
   b. Patients receiving oxygen
   c. Teenage patients
   d. Patients with broken ribs

6. Which patients should not have temperatures taken rectally?
   a. Patients with NG tubes
   b. Patients with diarrhea
   c. Infants
   d. Patients who smoke

7. How should a pulse be taken?
   a. With the first two or three fingers for about thirty seconds
   b. With the third and fourth finger on the femoral artery
   c. With the thumb on the jugular

d. With the thumb on the brachial artery

8. Which of the following counts as a respiration?
   a. An inhale
   b. An inhale and an exhale
   c. An exhale
   d. A cough

9. The apical pulse is taken:
   a. With the first and second finger
   b. Over the apex of the heart with the palm of the hand
   c. Over the apex of the heart with a stethoscope
   d. None of the above

10. The apical pulse is especially useful in:
    a. Infants or small children
    b. In the elderly
    c. In patients with brittle bones
    d. In patients going into fibrillation

11. When taking a pulse you should feel:
    a. On the radial artery which is located on the same side as the patient's pinky
    b. On the brachial artery on the back side of the arm
    c. On the temporal artery located on the forehead
    d. On the radial artery located on the same side as the patient's thumb

12. Tachypnea is characterized by:
    a. A rate of breathing greater than 40 breaths per minute
    b. A rate of breathing less than 10 breaths per minute
    c. A rate of breathing greater than 100 breaths per minute
    d. A rate of breathing less than 5 breaths per minute

13. A patient has a fever that has been fluctuating all day. However, the fever never returns to a baseline or a normal temperature. This is considered:
    a. Continuous fever
    b. Intermittent fever
    c. Remittent fever
    d. Afebrile fever

14. Apnea occurs when:
    a. The patient permanently stops breathing
    b. The patient temporarily has complete absence of breath
    c. The patient is in hysteria
    d. The patient is breathing normally

15. Bradypnea:
    a. Occurs when a patient hyperventilates
    b. Has a breathing rate of greater than 40 breaths per minute
    c. Is normal during a sleeping state
    d. Is never normal

16. Depth of respiration refers to:
    a. Number of breaths per minutes
    b. Amount of air inspired and expired
    c. Number of heartbeats per minute
    d. Amount of blood pumped through the heart per minute

17. Hypoventilation refers to a time when:
    a. Reduced air enters the lungs
    b. Increased air enters the lungs
    c. Normal amounts of air enters the lungs
    d. No air enters the lungs

18. Hypoventilation results in:
    a. Excess oxygen in the blood and decreased carbon dioxide in the blood
    b. Excess nitrogen in the blood and decreased carbon dioxide
    c. Decreased nitrogen in the blood and increased oxygen in the blood
    d. Decreased oxygen in the blood and increased carbon dioxide

19. Blood pressure can be described as:
    a. The distance pressurized blood will travel
    b. The amount of stress that veins can safely handle
    c. The amount of force exerted by blood on peripheral arteries
    d. None of the above

20. An instrument that measures blood pressure is known as a:
    a. Hypometer
    b. Sphygmomanometer
    c. Barometer
    d. Mercometer

21. Which artery does the blood pressure cuff center over?
    a. Jugular artery
    b. Femoral artery
    c. Antecubital artery
    d. Brachial artery

22. Failure to properly place the cuff can lead to:
    a. False diagnosis of high or low blood pressure
    b. Rupture of the veins
    c. Accurate diagnosis of high or low blood pressure

d. Discomfort

23. Cuffs that are too small or narrow can lead to:
    a. Unusually low blood pressure readings
    b. Abnormal heart rate readings
    c. Unusually high blood pressure readings
    d. All of the above

24. Anthropometric measurements refers to:
    a. Measurements of the heart and lungs
    b. Comparative measurements of the body
    c. Comparative measurements of lung function
    d. All of the above

25. During the examination, the medical assistant will be responsible for:
    a. Room and patient preparation
    b. Patient examination
    c. Patient treatment
    d. Room maintenance

26. Which of the following does the physician use to make a diagnosis?
    a. Patient history
    b. Lab tests
    c. Physical examination
    d. All of the above

27. How would someone examine a patient using palpation?
    a. Listening to breath sounds
    b. Tapping on a patient's chest to listen to the sounds
    c. Feeling a pulse
    d. All of the above

28. Which position is the most commonly used for patient examination?
    a. The vertical recumbent position
    b. The horizontal flat dorsal position
    c. Vertical pineal dorsal position
    d. The horizontal recumbent position

29. Which of the following is used for pelvic exams?
    a. Dorsal lithotomy position
    b. The horizontal recumbent position
    c. The vertical recumbent position
    d. Dilliad's position

30. A patient comes in for an exam. The patient is having trouble breathing. Which position do you place the patient in?

a. Vertical recumbent position
b. Fowler's position
c. Dilliard's position
d. Any of the above

31. Which position is used for a rectal exam?
    a. Fowler's position
    b. Prone position
    c. Sim's position
    d. Dilliard's position

32. Most accidents occur because:
    a. The patient does not cooperate
    b. Rules are overlooked or ignored
    c. Healthcare professionals don't care
    d. None of the above

33. Which of the following is an example of a hazard in the healthcare setting?
    a. Electrical hazards
    b. Biological hazards
    c. Chemical hazards
    d. All of the above

34. A coworker has noticed a stripped cord connected to a bed. This is an example of:
    a. Electrical hazards
    b. Biological hazards
    c. Chemical hazards
    d. Neurological hazards

35. Someone has left out some strong cleaning supplies. This is an example of:
    a. Electrical hazards
    b. Biological hazards
    c. Chemical hazards
    d. Neurological hazards

36. Someone has left out an uncapped, used sharp. This is an example of:
    a. Electrical hazards
    b. Biological hazards
    c. Chemical hazards
    d. Neurological hazards

37. A coworker has cut himself badly on a jagged piece of metal. You should:
    a. Have the coworker lie down
    b. Pour disinfectant on the wound
    c. Apply pressure and elevate the wound

d. Perform CPR

38. A patient is on the floor with cold/clammy skin, blank expression, and shallow breathing. This patient possibly is suffering from:
    a. Shock
    b. Stroke
    c. Heart attack
    d. Sun poisoning

39. CPR stands for:
    a. Cardio-Palpitative Resuscitation
    b. Carotid-Pulmonary Recognizance
    c. Cardio-Pulmonary Resuscitation
    d. Carotid-Palliative Recognizance

40. An influenza virus is an example of:
    a. An agent
    b. A portal of exit
    c. A mode of transmission
    d. A portal of entry

41. Which of the following is not an example of a portal of entry?
    a. A scratch on the hand
    b. Intact skin
    c. A mucous membrane
    d. Respiratory tract

42. Which of the following is not an example of a mode of transmission?
    a. Wearing gloves
    b. Being sneezed on
    c. Contact with blood
    d. Touching an infected surface

43. Which of the following means "the destruction of pathogenic microorganisms after they leave the body"?
    a. Vector transmission
    b. Asymmetry
    c. Medical Asepsis
    d. Organ Sepsis

44. When disinfecting items you should:
    a. Use chemicals on every item to be disinfected
    b. Put everything into a cleaning oven
    c. Wipe everything down with water
    d. Use chemicals only on inanimate objects

45. Which item would not be eligible to be cleaned with boiling water?
    a. An oral thermometer
    b. A pair of utility scissors
    c. A reflex hammer
    d. A mug

46. Surgical instruments are placed in an autoclave. This is an example of:
    a. Dry heat sterilization
    b. Chemical sterilization
    c. Steam sterilization
    d. Gas sterilization

47. A wheelchair is placed in a chamber for sterilization. This is most likely an example of:
    a. Dry heat sterilization
    b. Chemical sterilization
    c. Steam sterilization
    d. Gas sterilization

48. The most important way of fighting infection is:
    a. Dry heat sterilization
    b. Hand washing
    c. Cleaning things with bleach
    d. All of the above

49. You must wear a face shield for performing a procedure. This is an example of:
    a. Isolation
    b. Medical asepsis
    c. Barrier protection
    d. Contact asepsis

50. Standard precautions include which of the following?
    a. Wearing gloves
    b. Wearing face shields when necessary
    c. Disposing of sharps without recapping
    d. All of the above

51. In order to prevent airborne diseases from spreading you should use:
    a. Universal precautions
    b. Contact precautions
    c. Airborne precautions
    d. All of the above

52. You catch a cold after you drink after your daughter. This is an example of:
    a. Airborne contamination
    b. Indirect contact transmission
    c. Direct contact transmission

d. Vector transmission

53. A patient contracted a disease from the hospital. This is an example of:
    a. A nosocomial infection
    b. Direct contact transmission
    c. Barrier protection
    d. A susceptible host

54. A child develops a rash after playing closely with another child. This could be an example of:
    a. Direct contact transmission
    b. Airborne transmission
    c. Vector transmission
    d. Indirect contact transmission

55. A virus is an example of a:
    a. Susceptible host
    b. An agent
    c. A vector
    d. Portal of exit

56. Standard precautions are aimed at:
    a. Preventing the spread of infectious agents as they exit the reservoir
    b. Preventing the spread of infectious as they enter the susceptible host
    c. Preventing the spread of infectious agents as they travel through the air
    d. None of the above

57. When a person appears to be in shock you should:
    a. Have the person sit up and elevate the arms
    b. Have the person stand up and elevate the arms
    c. Have the person lay down and elevate the feet
    d. None of the above

58. When should you wash your hands?
    a. Before and after speaking with the patient
    b. Before and after entering a room
    c. After eating and using the bathroom
    d. After leaving the hospital

59. To avoid chemical hazards you should always:
    a. Store chemicals with non-hazardous materials
    b. Pour chemicals into clear bottles
    c. Label all chemicals with the MSDS
    d. All of the above

60. In order to avoid biological hazards you should:
    a. Incinerate any non-cleanable materials

b. Sterilize any materials that can be sterilized

c. Wash hands before and after each procedure

d. All of the above

61. To avoid electrical hazards you should:

a. Never use extension cords

b. Replace any cords that are bare or have the wire showing

c. Unplug electrical equipment before servicing

d. All of the above

62. When an accident occurs you should:

a. Attempt to clean up the mess before anyone notices

b. Talk about it with a co-worker

c. Report it to a supervisor

d. Leave it for someone else

63. A patient needs to be examined in the posterior aspect. Which position should you use for this patient?

a. Trendelenburg

b. Prone position

c. Sim's position

d. None of the above

64. Which of the following would a medical assistant do for the patient?

a. Collect vitals

b. Explain the procedure

c. Positioning and draping the patient

d. All of the above

65. Which of the following is not an anthropometric measurement?

a. Lucidity

b. Weight

c. Height

d. Head circumference

66. How fast should a blood pressure cuff deflate?

a. 1-2 mmHg per second

b. 2-3 mmHg per second

c. 4-5 mmHg per second

d. 6-7 mmHg per second

67. A state where increased air is entering the lungs is called:

a. Hypopnea

b. Hyperpnoea

c. Hyperventilation

d. Hypoventilation

68. Cheyne-Stokes refers to:
    a. Regular pattern of irregular breathing
    b. Irregular pattern of regular breathing
    c. Regular pattern of regular breathing
    d. Irregular pattern of irregular breathing

69. Orthopnea refers to:
    a. Trouble breathing because of problems with the rib bones
    b. Regular breathing in an inverted position
    c. Difficulty breathing when not upright
    d. Difficulty breathing when upright

70. Apnea refers to:
    a. A period of increased breathing, then returning to normal
    b. A period if no breath
    c. A period if decreased breath depth
    d. None of the above

71. When using a rectal thermometer:
    a. All patients are eligible for rectal thermometers
    b. Only babies should have rectal temperatures taken
    c. Only elderly patients should have rectal temperatures taken
    d. Patients with heart disease should not have rectal temperatures taken

72. If a patient has just been drinking or smoking you should:
    a. Take temperature orally anyway
    b. Wait thirty minutes and then take his/her temperature
    c. Wait ten minutes and then take temperature rectally
    d. None of the above

73. A patient is described as afebrile. This patient is:
    a. Having heart trouble
    b. Having breathing trouble
    c. Has a normal body temperature
    d. Has fertility problems

74. A patient has an axillary temperature of 98 degrees Fahrenheit. This patient:
    a. Has a normal body temperature
    b. Has a low body temperature
    c. Has a high body temperature
    d. Should be tested with an oral thermometer

75. Which of the following is not a place to take a temperature?
    a. Axillary area

b. Rectal area

c. Antecubital area

d. Ear

76. Social history includes:
    a. Summary of family health problems
    b. Lifestyle
    c. Past surgeries
    d. Chief complaint

77. Medical history includes:
    a. Past surgeries
    b. Major illnesses
    c. Medications
    d. All of the above

78. Family history includes:
    a. Health problems of parents
    b. Past surgeries
    c. Lifestyle
    d. Major illnesses

79. A systematic check of each organ and system along with documenting positive and negative results is called a:
    a. Review of the body
    b. Review of systems
    c. Review of the patient
    d. None of the above

80. A Medical Assistant might:
    a. Collect specimens
    b. Instruct a patient about medications
    c. Gather vitals
    d. All of the above

81. Medical assistants do not:
    a. Make a diagnosis
    b. Assist the physician
    c. Dispose of contaminated supplies
    d. Prepare patients for XRays

82. Medical assistants might:
    a. Do medical transcription
    b. Maintain medical records
    c. Manage finances

d. All of the above

83. An explanation of the chief complaint along with the symptoms and duration is part of:
    a. Social history
    b. Family history
    c. History of present illness
    d. Medical history

84. Which of the following is not a vital sign?
    a. Respiration
    b. Weight
    c. Pulse
    d. Temperature

85. Which of the following is the least accurate way to attain a temperature?
    a. Rectally
    b. Orally
    c. Ear
    d. Axillary

86. The normal pulse ranges between:
    a. 20 and 40 BPM
    b. 30 and 70 BPM
    c. 60 and 100 BPM
    d. 90 and 130 BPM

87. When taking a blood pressure with a stethoscope and a sphygmomanometer:
    a. Note the level at which two consecutive beats occur and the level at which all sounds disappear
    b. Note the level at which the blood pressure cuff becomes too tight
    c. Note the level at which the cuff completely deflates
    d. None of the above

88. To avoid biological hazards you should:
    a. Always wear gloves
    b. Disinfect the work area
    c. Wash hands
    d. All of the above

89. A person sneezes and germs are spread through drops across the room. This is an example of:
    a. Airborne transmission
    b. Droplet transmission
    c. Contact transmission
    d. All of the above

90. A person is blankly staring, has a rapid and weak pulse, and increased, shallow breathing. This person may be suffering from:
    a. Cheyne-Stokes
    b. Shock
    c. Stroke
    d. Hematoma

91. If it is necessary to use a bleach solution for disinfecting it should be diluted:
    a. 1 bleach : 1 water
    b. 2 bleach : 1 water
    c. 4 bleach : 1 water
    d. 1 bleach : 10 water

92. Airborne precautions are used to isolate:
    a. All patients that might have any contagion
    b. Any patients that might pose a direct contact threat
    c. Any patient that might offer airborne infection
    d. Only young and elderly patients

93. Contact precautions are used when:
    a. The patient might have a disease that is spread through direct contact
    b. A patient might have an airborne disease
    c. A patient might have a droplet disease
    d. None of the above

94. Standard precautions are:
    a. Precautions used only for contagious patients
    b. Precautions used only when the caregiver is ill
    c. Precautions used on all patients
    d. Precautions used only on foreign patients

95. Which of the following is the most important and most basic way of preventing disease transmission?
    a. Face masks
    b. Gloves
    c. Face shields
    d. Hand washing

96. Dry heat sterilization would be used for:
    a. Cleaning hands
    b. Cleaning wheelchairs
    c. Cleaning instruments that easily corrode
    d. Cleaning beds

97. A fungi is an example of a:
    a. Vector

b. Agent

c. Reservoir

d. Host

98. A person is bleeding. This is an example of:

a. Susceptible host

b. Shock

c. External hemorrhaging

d. All of the above

99. When should you wash your hands?

a. Before and after speaking with the patient

b. Before and after entering a room

c. After eating and using the bathroom

d. After leaving the hospital

100.   Which of the following pressurizes steam in order to sterilize?

a. Chemical sterilization

b. Dry heat sterilization

c. Steam sterilization

d. Water sterilization

Section One Answers

1. D
2. C
3. A
4. C
5. B
6. B
7. A
8. B
9. C
10. A
11. D
12. A
13. C
14. B
15. C
16. B
17. A
18. D
19. C
20. B
21. D

22. A
23. C
24. B
25. A
26. D
27. B
28. D
29. A
30. B
31. C
32. B
33. D
34. A
35. C
36. B
37. C
38. A
39. C
40. A
41. B
42. A
43. C
44. D
45. A
46. C
47. D
48. B
49. C
50. D
51. C
52. B
53. A
54. A
55. B
56. A
57. C
58. B
59. C
60. D
61. D
62. C
63. B
64. D
65. A
66. B
67. C

68. A
69. C
70. B
71. D
72. B
73. C
74. A
75. C
76. B
77. D
78. A
79. B
80. D
81. A
82. D
83. C
84. B
85. D
86. C
87. A
88. D
89. B
90. B
91. D
92. C
93. A
94. C
95. D
96. C
97. B
98. C
99. B
100.   C

Patient Care Procedures

Care of the surgical patient

A. Perform tasks from pre-operative checklist

    1. Showering, bathing

    2. Enemas - per hospital policy

    3. Nonsterile douche - per hospital policy

    4. Shave prep

    5. Hospital gown

    6. NPO after midnight or as ordered by physician

    7. Vital signs

    8. Remove dentures, if ordered.

    9. Remove prostheses (i.e., hearing aids, glasses, contact lenses, splints, braces, artificial parts).

    10. Remove jewelry, hair pins, makeup.

    11. Tape wedding rings, if allowed.

    12. Assure security of any items of value (i.e., give jewelry to family member with patient's permission).

    13. Have patient empty bladder. Drain Foley if present. Record output.

    14. Notify medication nurse when patient is ready.

    15. Provide for safe environment after pre-operative medication (i.e., side rails up, safety belt fastened on gurney, call light in reach).

B. Identify nurse assistant's role in pre-operational checklist

C. Document on the preoperative checklist

Nurse assistant's responsibilities while the patient is in surgery.

A. Prepare the room:

    1. Surgical bed

    2. Emesis basin

    3. Facial tissue

    4. Vital sign equipment

    5. IV pole

    6. Incontinent pads.

B. Collect additional equipment as ordered

    1. O_2 equipment

    2. Pulse Oximeter

    3. Suction

Patient care measures provided in the post-operative phase.

A. Post-operative checks

    1. Note time of return.

    2. Note level of consciousness.

    3. Check dressings for location and condition (dryness).

    4. Observe incisions, report any drainage, redness or swelling (assessing and changing the dressing is the responsibility of the licensed nurse).

    5. Check IV for location and observe site for redness, swelling, warmth or drainage.

    6. Observe to see that IV is dripping and tubing not kinked.

B. Post-operative care measures

    1. Assist in transfer from gurney to bed.

    2. Vital signs

        a. Be aware of changes in vital signs that signal hemorrhage, i.e., decreasing blood pressure and increasing pulse.

     b. Elevated temperature may signal infection.

     c. Report abnormalities to licensed personnel promptly.

     d. Pulse oximetry

  3. Observations

     a. Comfort: degree of pain or other discomfort

     b. Safety: side rails, call light within reach

     c. Equipment: report if disconnected or malfunctioning

     d. Changes in behavior: confusion, disorientation, agitation

     e. Changes in skin color: pallor, gray, blue-tinged

     f. Nausea, vomiting

     g. Bowel activity, passing gas

C. Care measures to prevent complications

  1. Encourage

     a. Turn, cough and deep breathing

     b. Incentive spirometer

     c. Leg exercises

  2. Apply TED hose and sequential compression de-vices, if ordered.

  3. Reposition at least every 2 hours to prevent hypo-static pneumonia.

  4. Apply binders, if ordered.

  5. Assist with dangling and initial ambulation, as ordered

  6. Review Hazards of Immobility and Role of the Nurse Assistant.

D. **Complications of Immobility: Deep Vein Thrombosis (DVT)** – blood clot in lower extremity

  1. General Information

     a. Deep vein thrombus (DVT) or blood clot occurs in pelvic veins or in deep veins of the lower extremities in post-operative patients. The incidence of DVT varies between 10% and 40% depending upon how serious the surgery is and how many other medical problems the patient has.

b. DVT is most common following hip surgery, then prostate surgery and general thoracic or abdominal surgery.

c. Blood clots located above the knee are considered the major source of pulmonary emboli (a blood clot that dislodges from the vein wall and travels to the lungs, causing death of lung tissue)

2. Causes

a. Pooling of blood in lower extremities (venous stasis)

b. Inactivity and immobility

c. Some medical conditions (stroke, heart attack, congestive heart failure)

d. Obesity

e. Varicose veins

f. Surgery and anesthesia

g. Age, particularly over 65 years

h. Damage to or stretching of blood vessels during surgery or trauma

i. Central venous catheters, pacemaker wires

j. Previous DVT

k. Increased tendency of blood to clot (some diseases like cancer, blood diseases, protein deficiency in malnourishment, dehydration)

l. Oral contraceptives and estrogen replacement

m. Smoking

3. Symptoms of DVT

a. Often have no symptoms

b. Pain or cramp in the calf or thigh, progressing to painful swelling of entire leg

c. Slight fever, chills, perspiration (diaphoresis), generalized feeling of discomfort

d. Painful tenderness over inner thigh

4. Prevention

a. Increased activity, early ambulation after surgery, frequent and proper repositioning

b. Range of motion

  c. Anti-embolic stockings (TED hose)

  d. Purpose of anti-embolic stockings

    1) To help prevent formation of blood clots

    2) To promote increased blood flow in the legs by compression of deep veins

    3) To improve venous return from the legs to the heart maintenance of anti-embolic stockings

    4) Properly sized stockings need to be removed daily during bathing to inspect condition of skin. Do not leave off more than 30 minutes.

    5) Wash stockings every 2 to 3 days to remove bodily secretions.

    6) For patient's information at home, the stockings can usually be machine washed on delicate and machine dried on low for 15 to 20 minutes.

    7) With correct care stockings last 3 to 4 months.

    8) Do not use ointments on the leg when using anti-embolic stockings.

  e. Sequential compressions sleeves or devices

  f. Adequate fluids

  g. Avoid dependent positioning of lower extremities (elevate legs when up in chair, avoid knee gatch when in bed).

  h. Doctor may order anticoagulants for licensed nurse to administer; observe for signs of bleeding or bruising.

  i. Observe for pain in calf, fever or chills, painful swelling of leg, tenderness over inner thigh.

  j. Report any shortness of breath or chest pain immediately to the licensed nurse.

E. *Nursing Alert*

 1. *A complaint of slight soreness of the calf is never ignored. Blood clots in the calf or thigh can break loose and travel to the lungs (pulmonary embolism). This is life threatening.*

 2. *Close observation of patients and attention to their complaints of pain or discomfort is very important.*

 3. *Report this to the licensed nurse.*

 4. *Never rub or massage the lower legs.*

SEQUENTIAL COMPRESSION DEVICES

Several types of devices are available that supply intermittent compression over the lower leg, thigh or foot. Each device aids in the return of venous blood and helps prevent deep vein thrombosis and pulmonary embolism. They are usually used in addition to anti-embolic stockings.

The typical type of sequential compression device consists of a vinyl or plastic sleeve that fits over the foot, lower leg or thigh. It may come as a tube or as a wrap style that fastens with Velcro. It is attached to a control unit that is placed on the floor under the bed. The control unit has a small pump that inflates and deflates channels in the sleeve to provide increasing and decreasing pressure. Connecting tubing attaches to the sleeve and to the control unit completing a closed system. The pressure can be adjusted according to facility policy or as ordered by the physician.

The device should be removed at least twice daily for 20 to 30 minutes to allow for ambulation, bathing and inspection of the skin. Sequential compression devices are usually worn at least 3 days after surgery or until the patient is up and ambulating regularly or as long as the doctor orders.

EQUIPMENT:

1. Sequential compression sleeves
2. Connectors
3. Control unit

CRITERIA:

Safely cares for the patient on a sequential compression device

1. Wash hands, identify patient, introduce self, explain procedure and provide for privacy.

2. Position patient, exposing one leg at a time for application of sequential sleeve.

3. Align leg on the open sleeve according to instructions included in package.

4. Wrap the sleeve securely around the patient's leg and fasten the Velcro tabs, thigh section first. Make sure that no wrinkles are in the plastic of the sleeve and that at least two fingers can be inserted between the patient's leg and the sleeve.

5. Make sure the control unit is turned off.

6. Attach the connector on the sleeve to the correct end of the connector tubing. Check carefully to be certain there are no kinks or twists in the tubing.

7. Attach the other end of the connector tubing to the control unit.

8. Turn the power on and adjust or monitor the pressure according to your facility's policy.

9. Remain with the patient for at least a complete cycle to monitor comfort and the functioning of the unit.

10. Sleeves should be removed if the patient experiences numbness, tingling or leg pain. Notify licensed nurse if any of these symptoms occur.

11. Document time of application, type of device, condition of skin and comfort of patient.

PRECAUTIONS:

1. Do not apply to any patient experiencing skin rash or poor circulation evidenced by bluish-red coloring of lower legs and feet, sores on lower legs or feet, severe edema or leg pain, edema of the lungs from congestive heart failure.

2. Make sure that connectors and sleeves are properly applied.

3. Monitor the patient's condition frequently, according to facility policy.

SINGLE LEG APPLICATION:

1. Most brands of sequential compression devices can be used on only one leg, if necessary.

2. The unused sleeve is kept in the plastic wrapper and attached to the second sleeve connector.

3. The compression action of the pump will not work unless there is a closed system. By keeping the unused sleeve folded in the wrapper, the system will be able to reach the proper compression.

MEASURING AND APPLICATION OF ANTI-EMBOLIC STOCKINGS

EQUIPMENT:

1. Tape measure (new one for each patient)

2. Scratch pad, order form or requisition form from Central Supply

3. Anti-embolic stockings (TED stockings or other brands)

CRITERIA:

Correctly measures and applies anti-embolic stockings

A. Thigh length

    1. Measure upper thigh circumference at gluteal furrow.

    2. Measure calf circumference at widest area.

    3. Measure length from gluteal furrow to base of heel.

    4. Consult sizing chart from Central Supply or TED stockings order pad, if available.

       ○ TED thigh length with belt stocking fit a thigh circumference of up to 32 inches.

       ○ TED thigh length stocking fit a maximum thigh circumference of 25 inches.

B. Knee length

    1. Measure calf circumference at widest area.

2. Measure length from bend of knee to base of heel.

C. Medicare usually covers two pair to insure that compression goes uninterrupted during laundering care. Check with the RN to see if one or two pair should be ordered.

D. Different brands of anti-embolic elastic stockings are available. Each pair will have a large round hole in the toe to check for circulation. In some brands the hole will be on top of the toes and some will have the hole open under the toes.

APPLICATION OF ANTI-EMBOLIC STOCKINGS:

1. Obtain correct size of anti-embolic stockings.
2. Wash hands, identify patient, introduce self, explain procedure and provide for privacy.
3. With patient lying down, expose one leg at a time for application of stocking.
4. Insert hand into stocking as far as the heel pocket.
5. Grasp center of heel pocket and turn stocking inside out to heel area.
6. Position stocking over foot and heel. Be sure patient's heel is centered in heel pocket.
7. Pull a few inches of the stocking up around the ankle and calf.
8. Continue pulling the stocking up the leg. If there is a change in the sheerness of the stocking material, it should fall between 1" to 2" below the bend of the knee.
9. As thigh portion of the stocking is applied, start rotating stocking inward so gusset is centered over femoral artery. Gusset is placed slightly towards the inside of the leg. When using thigh length stockings, the top band rests in the gluteal furrow.
10. Smooth out wrinkles.

11. Align inspection toe to fall at base of toes either on the top or underneath, depending on brand.
12. Instruct patient on proper positioning of stockings to insure that he/she will not reposition the stockings incorrectly.
13. Repeat procedure on opposite leg.

14. Wash hands.

15. Report procedure and document size and style of stocking applied.

16. Document when stockings are removed along with condition of skin.

17. Report any tenderness in calves, thighs or toes.

TURNING A SURGICAL PATIENT

EQUIPMENT:

1. Pillows

2. Lift sheet

CRITERIA:

Safely turns a surgical patient

Instruct patient in splinting incision for comfort.

1. Obtain patient activity orders from licensed nurse.

2. Instruct patient in splinting incision for comfort.

3. Make sure that bed wheels are locked, curtains are pulled around bed for privacy and bed is raised to highest level for good body mechanics.

4. Lower head of bed if patient's condition allows.

5. Using good body mechanics, turn patient.

6. Position patient for comfort and in good body alignment.

    a. Place pillow under head.

    b. Position a pillow against back for support.

    c. Place a pillow in front of the bottom leg and place the top leg on top of the pillow in a flexed position.

    d. Check lower shoulder to make sure it is not squeezed in an abnormal position. Reach under shoulder and pull forward gently until patient is comfortable.

  e. Support upper arm and hand with a pillow for comfort, either in front of the

   patient or back on the pillow behind the patient.

  f. If abdominal incision is pulling, may place pillow under side of abdomen.

7. Place the signal cord within reach; raise side rails, lower bed to lowest position, open curtains

  around bed.

DANGLE AND AMBULATE A SURGICAL PATIENT

CRITERIA:

Safely dangles and ambulates a surgical patient

---

1. Check patient's pulse, blood pressure and respirations.

2. Assist patient to side of bed and put on non-slip slippers.

3. Assist patient to pivot and sit at side of bed.

4. Support patient and observe for abnormal signs.

5. Assist patient to put on robe.

6. Apply gait belt if allowed.

7. Assist the patient to stand.

8. Stand at patient's side until steady, holding the gait belt in the middle of the patient's back.

9. Stand slightly behind patient, on weak side, if applicable.

10. Encourage patient to walk with head up, standing erect.

11. Observe for signs of activity intolerance (increased pain, shortness of breath,

   pallor, diaphoresis).

12. Return patient to bed and make sure patient is safe and comfortable.

13. Report distance patient walked and how well patient tolerated activity to licensed

nurse.

14. If patient has an IV, may need two people to assist with ambulation.

HAZARDS OF IMMOBILITY AND ROLE OF THE NURSE ASSISTANT

1.   Cardiovascular complications - blood clots, orthostatic hypotension, increased work on the heart

- Remind patient to do exercises given by the physical and occupational therapist.

  - Encourage intake of adequate fluids to prevent dehydration.

  - Early ambulation as allowed.

  - Proper positioning and avoidance of pressure on blood vessels.

  - Do not massage the calf of the leg.

2.   Respiratory complications – slow and shallow respirations, pooling of respiratory secretions, hypostatic pneumonia, pulmonary embolism

  - Remind patient to turn, cough, take deep breaths and to use incentive spirometer.

  - Increase activity as soon as allowed by patient's condition and doctor's orders.

  - Encourage fluids as allowed to keep lung secretions thinned.

3.   Gastrointestinal complications – poor appetite, poor nutrition, constipation, fecal impaction

- Offer adequate fluids.

  - Prevent incontinence by timely offering of the bedpan and early mobility for access to the bathroom.

  - Monitor patient's appetite and ask RN to assess need for a dietician consult.

4.   Urinary system complications – urinary retention, incontinence, increased risk of kidney stones, urinary tract infections

- Keep accurate record of intake and output.

- Observe for pain in the back and blood in the urine.

- Observe for signs of urinary tract infection: pain with urination, frequent urination of small amounts, feeling the need to urinate all the time, concentrated or cloudy urine.

5. Musculoskeletal system complications – muscle wasting and atrophy, stiff joints, decreased balance, loss of endurance, osteoporosis, contractures, foot drop

- Perform passive ROM exercises for patients who are unable to do them, and instruct patients who are able to do active or active-assistive ROM.

- Position patients properly in bed, using good body alignment.

- Remind and reinforce any exercises given to patient by physical or occupational therapists and RN.

6. Integumentary system complications – pressure on bony prominences, impaired circulation to skin layers, skin breakdown, pressure ulcers, infections

- Observe for any sign of redness or sores on the skin.

- Keep skin clean and dry.

- Keep bedding free of wrinkles and crumbs.

- Turn patient at least every 2 hours to reduce pressure on bony prominence

Gastro-intestinal care

Common diseases/disorders of the GI system.

A. Congenital: cleft palate

B. Inflammation: stomatitis, esophagitis, gastro-enteritis, colitis, cholecystitis, pancreatitis, hepatitis, cholelithiasis

C. Ulceration: stomach, duodenum, colon

D. Hernias: inguinal, umbilical, hiatal, inicisional.

E. Tumors: benign, malignant

F. Bowel disorders: distension, diarrhea, constipation, and impaction

Patient preparation for GI diagnostic tests.

    A. Radiology Testing

        1. UGI

        2. Small bowel series

        3. Gall bladder series

        4. Barium enema

    B. Direct Visualization

        1. Colonoscopy/sigmoidoscopy

        2. Esophagogastroduodenoscopy (EGD)

        3. Gastroscopy

        4. Endoscopy

        5. Swallowing evaluation

        6. Gastric sampling

        7. Ultrasound

    C. Preparing the patient for diagnostic tests

        1. NPO for at least eight hours (or as ordered)

        2. Give enemas as ordered.

        3. Laxatives given by licensed nurse as ordered.

Special diets as ordered

    A. Purpose of enemas: to aid in illumination during x-rays, before surgery, before deliveries, before direct visualization tests, for bowel retraining, to relieve constipation, to expel flatus, to instill medicine.

B. Types of enemas

    1. Cleansing: SSE, TWE, saline, Fleet's phosphosoda.

    2. Retention: medicinal, nutritional, Fleet's oil retention.

    3. Return Flow: Harris flush (HF).

A. Purpose of the sitz bath.

    1. Cleansing

    2. Heat

Healing after perineal/rectal surgery or infant delivery

A. Abnormal signs and symptoms to report to licensed nurse.

    1. Weakness

    2. Rapid, weak pulse

    3. Low blood pressure

    4. Rapid or labored respirations

    5. Fatigue

    6. Dizziness

    7. Fainting

    8. Bleeding (coffee grounds emesis, black, tarry stools, rectal bleeding)

    9. Change in drainage

    10. Change in stool

The difference in care measures between hemodialysis and peritoneal dialysis.

A. Hemodialysis:

    1. Procedure that filters and cleans waste products from the blood. It is performed by specially trained RNs.

2. Never take blood pressure in arm with a fistula or shunt

B. Peritoneal dialysis:

   1. Removes extra water, waste, and chemicals from body by perfusing sterile solutions through the peritoneal cavity and using the thin membrane that lines the abdominal organs, (peritoneum) as a filter. The dialyzed solution drains out through an abdominal tube.

   2. Reporting abnormal signs and symptoms

      a. Fever, nausea/vomiting

      b. Abdominal pain

      c. Redness around the catheter

      d. Change in vital signs

   3. Special considerations - no ointments or powder around peritoneal catheter.

   4. Prevention of infection

   5. Standard precautions

Reproductive system care

The common sexually transmitted diseases (STDs).

A. Syphilis

B. Gonorrhea

C. Herpes simplex

D. Venereal warts

E. AIDS

F. Chlamydia

   1. Method of transmission:

      a. Mucous membrane to mucous membrane

      b. Mucous membrane to skin

      c. Skin to mucous membrane

2. Stress nursing considerations: importance of treating all patients with respect and avoiding judgmental attitude regarding patient's lifestyle.

Care measures for the postpartum patient.

   A. Observe vaginal discharge for color/odor

      1. Lochia rubra: dark or bright red 3-4 days

      2. Lochia serosa: pinkish brown 10 days

      3. Lochia alba: whitish 2-6 weeks

   B. Report number of pads used

   C. Observe perineal area for signs of infection

   D. Set up sitz bath

   E. Assist mom with breastfeeding

   F. Watch for signs of urine retention

   G. Report bowel activity

   H. Burning on urination

   I. Leg pain, tenderness, swelling

   J. Sadness or feelings of depression

   K. Breast pain, tenderness, swelling

Reportable signs and symptoms of postpartum complications.

   A. Fever

   B. Abdominal or perineal pain

   C. Foul smelling vaginal discharge

   D. Bleeding from episiotomy or c-section incision

   E. Redness/swelling or drainage from c-section incision

   F. Saturating sanitary napkin within one hour of application

   G. Red lochia after changed to brown

GOOD LUCK IN YOUR EXAMS!!!

www.ingramcontent.com/pod-product-compliance
Lightning Source LLC
Chambersburg PA
CBHW081224170526
45165CB00009B/2940